HEART HEALTH HARMONY

Revolutionary Therapies For
Cardiovascular Wellness

Explore Groundbreaking Therapies For Heart Health And Unlock The Secrets To A Strong And Resilient Cardiovascular System

DR. BRIDGET PROMISE

Table of Contents

CHAPTER ONE

Introduction

Cardiovascular health is an important part of general well-being since it helps to prolong life and vigor. Understanding the complexities of cardiovascular health entails investigating the different components that contribute to its optimal functioning or, conversely, degeneration.

This in-depth talk looks into the world of cardiovascular health, highlighting the importance of lifestyle choices, breakthrough treatments, and the mind-body link in supporting a strong and resilient heart.

Understanding Cardiovascular Health

At its core, cardiovascular health refers to the status of the heart and blood arteries, which form the cardiovascular system. A healthy cardiovascular system supports proper blood circulation, giving oxygen and nutrients to cells while eliminating waste items.

Understanding the essential components of cardiovascular health requires knowledge of both the heart's anatomy and physiological functioning.

The heart, a muscular organ, circulates blood via a network of blood vessels that includes arteries, veins, and capillaries. Arteries convey oxygenated blood from the heart to other areas of the body, whereas veins return deoxygenated blood to the heart.

Capillaries are microscopic blood arteries that promote the passage of nutrients and oxygen between the blood and tissues.

Maintaining cardiovascular health is critical for avoiding illnesses including heart disease, stroke, and hypertension. Individuals' cardiovascular well-being is influenced by their lifestyle choices, genetics, and environmental circumstances.

The Role Of Lifestyle In Heart Health:

Lifestyle decisions have a substantial impact on cardiovascular health. Adopting a heart-healthy lifestyle may lower the risk of cardiovascular disease and improve overall well-being. A balanced diet, frequent physical exercise, stress management, and abstaining from dangerous behaviors like smoking are all important components of a heart-healthy lifestyle.

A well-balanced diet is essential for maintaining cardiovascular health. Fruits, vegetables, healthy grains, and lean proteins should be prioritized above saturated fats, cholesterol, and salt to promote good heart health. Maintaining a healthy weight is particularly important since obesity is a recognized risk factor for heart disease.

Regular physical exercise is another key component of heart health. Exercise strengthens the heart muscle, boosts blood circulation, and aids in weight management. Aerobic workouts such as walking, running, or cycling improve cardiovascular endurance, while strength training helps with overall fitness.

Stress management is very important for cardiovascular health. Chronic stress may lead to hypertension and other cardiovascular problems. Incorporating relaxation practices like meditation, deep breathing exercises, or yoga into one's daily routine may help to reduce the detrimental effects of stress on the heart.

CHAPTER TWO

Revolutionary Therapies Overview

Medical advances have cleared the door for ground-breaking medicines to address cardiovascular ailments. These treatments, which vary from breakthrough drugs to cutting-edge surgical techniques, provide fresh hope for those dealing with cardiac problems.

Statins, antiplatelet medicines, and beta-blockers are typical medications used to lower cholesterol, prevent blood clots, and control blood pressure. These medicinal therapies, when paired with lifestyle changes, may considerably lower the risk of cardiovascular disease.

Invasive treatments, such as angioplasty and coronary artery bypass grafting (CABG), are used to treat more severe forms of cardiovascular disease.

Angioplasty involves inserting a catheter to expand constricted arteries, while CABG reroutes blood flow around blocked arteries via grafts. These therapies seek to restore normal blood flow to the heart, therefore relieving symptoms and enhancing overall cardiac performance.

Emerging medicines, such as gene therapy and stem cell treatments, provide promise for healing damaged cardiac tissue and boosting regeneration. These revolutionary technologies have the potential to transform cardiovascular therapy by tackling the underlying causes of heart disease at the genetic and cellular levels.

Mind-Body Connections And Heart Health

The mind-body link is critical for cardiovascular health, yet it is frequently overlooked. Mental and emotional well-being may influence heart function, contributing to the development or prevention of cardiovascular disease.

Chronic stress, worry, and depression all raise the chance of developing heart disease. Stress hormones generated during times of high stress may cause higher blood pressure, inflammation, and changes in blood coagulation, all of which have a detrimental influence on cardiovascular health. Thus, developing mental and emotional resilience is critical for sustaining a healthy heart.

Mind-body techniques such as meditation, mindfulness, and yoga are helpful tools for stress management and emotional well-being. These behaviors not only lower stress, but also benefit heart health by reducing blood pressure, heart rate variability, and overall cardiac function.

To summarize, understanding cardiovascular health requires a comprehensive approach that includes the anatomical and physiological elements of the heart, the influence of lifestyle choices, new therapeutics, and the delicate relationship between the mind and body. Individuals may take proactive actions to ensure the longevity and vibrancy of their cardiovascular system by adopting a heart-healthy lifestyle, using novel treatments, and understanding the value of mental and emotional well-being.

Maintaining cardiovascular health is critical for general well-being, and implementing dietary recommendations, regular exercise, stress reduction methods, and prioritizing excellent sleep may all help to promote cardiovascular harmony.

Dietary Strategies For Cardiovascular Harmony

A heart-healthy diet is essential for maintaining good cardiovascular health. Consuming nutrient-dense meals while minimizing saturated fats, cholesterol, and salt may have a major influence on heart health. A diet rich in fruits, vegetables, whole grains, and lean meats contains important nutrients and fiber.

The Mediterranean diet, known for its cardiovascular advantages, contains olive oil, seafood, nuts, and seeds, demonstrating the importance of eating good fats.

Reducing processed foods and sugar consumption aids in weight management and lowers the chance of acquiring disorders such as obesity and diabetes, both of which are associated with cardiovascular disease. Furthermore, eating foods rich in omega-3 fatty acids, such as salmon and mackerel, helps to reduce inflammation and promotes heart health.

Monitoring portion sizes is another critical component of a heart-healthy diet. Overeating may cause weight growth, increasing the pressure on the heart. Using smaller dishes, being conscious of portion sizes, and responding to hunger signals are all useful ways.

Exercise is a pillar of heart health.

Regular physical exercise is an essential component of cardiovascular health. Aerobic workouts like brisk walking, jogging, cycling, and swimming help to strengthen the heart and improve circulation. The American Heart Association advises at least 150 minutes of moderate-intensity activity or 75 minutes of strenuous exercise every week for good cardiovascular health.

Exercise not only helps you maintain a healthy weight, but it also has a favorable effect on your cholesterol, blood pressure, and blood sugar. It also enhances the effective working of the heart, increasing its capacity to pump blood throughout the body.

Strength training activities at least two days per week improve heart health by increasing muscle mass, which may help with weight management and overall cardiovascular fitness. A balanced approach to exercise includes cardiovascular activities, strength training, and flexibility exercises.

CHAPTER THREE

Holistic Approaches To Stress Reduction

Stress, whether chronic or acute, has a deleterious influence on cardiovascular health. Taking a comprehensive approach to stress reduction is critical for reaching cardiovascular harmony. Meditation, deep breathing exercises, and mindfulness are helpful stress-reduction techniques.

Yoga, which emphasizes breath control, meditation, and moderate exercise, has been demonstrated to lower stress and enhance cardiovascular health. Regular yoga practice may help to lower blood pressure, reduce heart rate, and enhance general mental well-being.

Stress management relies heavily on social ties and emotional support. Building and sustaining solid connections with friends and family may provide you with a feeling of belonging and security, lessening the detrimental effects of stress on your heart.

Optimize Your Sleep For A Healthy Heart

Quality sleep is sometimes disregarded, although it is critical to preserving cardiovascular health. Sleep deprivation may cause a variety of complications, including an increased risk of hypertension, obesity, and diabetes, all of which contribute to heart disease.

Establishing a regular sleep schedule, aiming for 7-9 hours of sleep every night, and establishing a sleep-friendly atmosphere are all critical for improving sleep. Avoiding stimulants like coffee close to bedtime, minimizing screen time before sleep, and creating a pleasant sleep environment all help to ensure a good night's sleep.

Sleep problems, including sleep apnea, may influence heart health. Seeking expert treatment if sleep difficulties continue is critical for treating any underlying concerns and improving overall cardiovascular health.

To summarize, establishing cardiovascular harmony requires a comprehensive strategy that includes dietary recommendations, regular exercise, stress reduction measures, and prioritizing sound sleep. Individuals may help avoid cardiovascular disease and maintain overall heart health by eating a heart-healthy diet rich in nutrient-dense foods, exercising regularly, reducing stress with holistic practices, and optimizing sleep. These lifestyle choices not only benefit the heart but also lead to better mental health and quality of life. Individuals who adopt these techniques empower themselves to take control of their cardiovascular health and improve their overall vitality.

Community And Social Connection

In the complex web of variables impacting cardiovascular health, community, and social connectedness emerge as a major influencer. As we explore more into the interrelated realms of heart health, it becomes clear that the support systems, connections, and community ties we cultivate play an important role in sustaining and improving cardiovascular health.

The value of true social ties cannot be emphasized in today's fast-paced world. Numerous research have examined the effects of social isolation and loneliness on cardiovascular health. Individuals without a strong social network may suffer higher amounts of stress, increasing their risk of heart disease. In contrast, people who live in supportive communities had better heart health results.

Communities serve as a buffer against the stresses of everyday life. Individuals discover ways to relieve stress, whether via shared physical activity, communal events, or just having a solid social group. Chronic stress has been linked to an increased risk of cardiovascular disease, and community participation may help to alleviate its negative consequences.

Furthermore, the community component goes beyond emotional support and includes lifestyle considerations. Communities often exchange resources and knowledge, which influences the adoption of heart-healthy habits. From community fitness programs to group cooking courses focusing on heart-healthy foods, the collaborative effort to promote cardiovascular wellness generates an atmosphere favorable to healthier living.

Herbal Allies for Cardiovascular Support, Exploring the Power of Supplements, Integrative Practices, Mindful Practices for Heart-Centered Living, and

Cultivating Emotional Resilience are examples of innovative medicinal approaches.

As our awareness of holistic well-being grows, so do creative pharmacological approaches to cardiovascular health. The combination of standard and alternative therapies has cleared the path for a more comprehensive approach to cardiovascular health.

This comprehensive approach includes herbal allies, supplements, integrative techniques, mindful living, and emotional resilience, all of which contribute to improved cardiovascular health.

Nature has historically provided healing, and herbal allies play an important role in improving cardiovascular health. Traditional herbal medicines, including hawthorn, garlic, and ginkgo biloba, have been shown to improve cardiac function. Hawthorn, for example, has been used for millennia to improve cardiovascular circulation, while garlic is thought to help maintain healthy blood pressure. Ginkgo biloba is another plant recognized for its antioxidant capabilities, which may help to preserve blood vessels.

These herbal friends are often ingested in a variety of formats, such as teas, tinctures, or capsules, enabling people to smoothly integrate them into their daily routines. The combination of these herbs may give a natural and mild approach to cardiovascular support, supplementing traditional medical therapies.

Exploring the Power of Supplements: Supplements have emerged as an important tool in the search for heart health. Omega-3 fatty acids, obtained from fish oil, are well known for their cardiovascular advantages. These important fatty acids help to reduce inflammation and may promote overall heart health. Another supplement that has been researched for its ability to sustain cardiovascular function is coenzyme Q10 (CoQ10), which is an antioxidant.

Vitamins such as B-complex vitamins, notably B6, B12, and folic acid, are essential for homocysteine metabolism, an amino acid associated with heart health. Furthermore, magnesium and potassium supplements may help to maintain normal blood pressure levels. While it is important to speak with healthcare specialists before introducing supplements, their importance in maintaining cardiovascular health should not be underestimated.

Integrative Practices and Heart Wellness: The combination of traditional and alternative medicine has resulted in integrative practices that seek to offer a comprehensive approach to heart health. Integrative medicine integrates evidence-based medical procedures with complementary treatments to provide a holistic and patient-centered approach to healthcare.

Mind-body therapies like yoga and tai chi have been recognized for their beneficial effects on cardiovascular health. These activities not only improve physical fitness but also help to reduce stress, which is important for heart health. Acupuncture, an ancient Chinese therapy, is another integrative method that has shown potential for improving cardiovascular function.

Nutritional therapies, informed by both ancient knowledge and current science, are an essential component of integrative approaches. A heart-healthy diet high in fruits, vegetables, whole grains, and lean meats promotes general cardiovascular health. The collaborative aspect of integrative treatments allows people to actively engage in their health journey, which fosters a feeling of empowerment.

Mindful Practices for Heart-Centered Living: Mindfulness, which is based on ancient contemplative practices, has received a lot of attention for its beneficial effects on heart health. Mindful techniques, such as meditation and deep breathing exercises, help to reduce stress and improve emotional well-being. Chronic stress has been related to cardiovascular problems, and mindfulness training may be a useful strategy for stress management.

Mindful eating, an extension of mindfulness, helps people to enjoy and appreciate their meals, resulting in a healthy relationship with food. Awareness of food choices and eating habits benefits overall heart health by encouraging a balanced diet and minimizing overindulgence in harmful foods.

Cultivating Emotional Resilience: The capacity to adapt and recover from life's adversities is an essential component of heart health. The delicate relationship between emotional well-being and cardiovascular health emphasizes the need to develop resilience. Practices like gratitude writing, positive affirmations, and hobbies may all help you feel better emotionally.

Emotional resilience relies heavily on social ties and supportive relationships. Maintaining good interpersonal interactions and seeking assistance when necessary help to build a strong emotional foundation. Furthermore, mental health treatments such as therapy and counseling help people negotiate emotional issues, which improves their heart health.

Finally, the study of novel pharmaceutical treatments in cardiovascular health requires a comprehensive framework. Herbal allies, supplements, integrative techniques, mindfulness, and emotional resilience all contribute to a holistic plan for heart health. Individuals who embrace these techniques may actively engage in their health journey, promoting a healthy and robust cardiovascular system.

CHAPTER FOUR

Environmental Factors And Cardiovascular Wellness

As we investigate the multidimensional terrain of cardiovascular health, the role of environmental variables becomes an important concern.

Our surroundings, including the air we breathe and the locations we live in, may have a substantial impact on our heart health results. Recognizing and managing these environmental influences is critical to maintaining a heart-healthy lifestyle.

Air quality, a key environmental component, has been related to cardiovascular disease. Air pollutants including particulate matter and ozone may cause inflammation and oxidative stress, both of which can lead to cardiac problems.

Urban surroundings, which are often characterized by increased pollution levels, provide extra difficulties to cardiovascular health. Implementing policies and personal habits that limit air pollution is critical for preserving heart health at both the individual and community levels.

The built environment, which includes neighborhood walkability and access to green areas, is also important. Communities with sidewalks, parks, and recreational places increase physical exercise and contribute to overall cardiovascular health.

These surroundings promote regular exercise, a critical component of heart health, by making it more accessible and enjoyable to people.

Furthermore, the job environment might impact cardiovascular health. Sedentary jobs and stressful work environments lead to a less heart-healthy lifestyle. Encouraging workplace activities that encourage physical exercise, stress management, and a heart-conscious culture may improve workers' cardiovascular health.

Personalized Heart Health Plans

In the goal of total cardiovascular fitness, the paradigm is evolving toward individualized health regimens. Recognizing the specific genetic, behavioral, and environmental variables that influence a person's heart health enables focused and successful preventative and treatment interventions.

Personalized heart health programs include a comprehensive evaluation of a person's risk factors. Tailored therapies are developed by taking into account genetic predispositions, family history, and lifestyle choices. Advances in genetic testing enable healthcare providers to detect particular genetic markers linked to cardiovascular risk, allowing for more individualized diet, exercise, and lifestyle advice.

Dietary preferences and sensitivities are important aspects of individualized heart health strategies. While broad dietary recommendations for heart health exist, personalized nutritional counsel improves adherence and efficacy. A tailored approach takes into account an individual's cultural background, culinary preferences, and any pre-existing health concerns to ensure that dietary recommendations are appropriate for their lifestyle.

Physical exercise, a key component of cardiovascular well-being, is also tailored to an individual's fitness level, preferences, and any current health issues. From personalized exercise routines to adaptive fitness programs, the objective is to make physical activity fun and sustainable, promoting long-term commitment.

Patient Success Stories

In the story of cardiovascular health, patient success stories serve as sources of inspiration and encouragement. These tales shed light on the transforming journeys people take to reclaim control of their heart health, offering hope and useful insights to others suffering similar issues.

Patient success stories include a wide range of experiences, from overcoming lifestyle risks to managing difficult medical procedures. These tales often emphasize the importance of community support, individualized health regimens, and human resilience.

Many success stories demonstrate the benefits of lifestyle adjustments for heart health. Individuals who have adopted better diets participated in regular physical exercise, and successfully handled stress share their stories to demonstrate the transforming potential of lifestyle changes. These experiences serve as useful guidance for those who want to take similar steps toward improved heart health.

When medical treatments are involved, patient success stories highlight the necessity of tailored care regimens. Whether it's a successful heart surgery, a well-managed recovery from a cardiac incident, or good medication management, these tales highlight the need for a comprehensive and personalized approach to cardiovascular health.

CHAPTER FIVE

Conclusion: A Heart-Healthy Future.

Finally, achieving cardiovascular wellness requires a dynamic interplay of community and social relationships, environmental concerns, tailored health programs, and inspiring patient success stories. As we manage the intricacies of contemporary life, we must acknowledge the combined influence of these variables on heart health.

Fostering strong community bonds and social relationships helps people handle life's obstacles, reduces stress, and promotes heart health. Environmental elements, ranging from air quality to the architecture of our living spaces, have a substantial impact on cardiovascular outcomes, highlighting the necessity of sustainable and heart-healthy environmental practices.

Personalized heart health programs represent a paradigm shift toward precision medicine by recognizing the unique character of cardiovascular risk factors. Healthcare practitioners may improve the efficacy of preventative programs and treatment plans by adapting treatments to the specific traits and preferences of each client.

Patient success stories serve as guiding beacons, demonstrating the transforming power of adopting heart-healthy habits and navigating personalized treatment programs. These stories instill hope, perseverance, and a feeling of agency in those aiming for improved heart health.

To imagine a heart-healthy future, it is critical to continue cultivating supportive communities, pushing for sustainable environmental practices, and adopting tailored approaches to cardiovascular wellness. Through our combined efforts, we may envision a future in which heart health is prioritized, celebrated, and accessible to everyone, leading to a society in which people flourish with healthy hearts and robust well-being.